THE #1 METHOD TO BURN BODY FAT

An Easy & Rapid Weight Loss Book MurderLoss

Nouhou Tambwe

CONTENTS

You have landed in the right spot, and I think it is amazing that you share a common interest with me... The fact that you want to lose weight, be healthy, and completely change your lifestyle for the better. As for myself, my journey really started when I was twelve years old. I was returning from school one day, and as my dad drove us through the school gates, he looked at me, and said: "You must get used to walking home after school, because I may not be there for you all the time. My health conditions are getting very bad, and your mum is unwell too. ' After hearing these words, I had horrible feelings that *I was not good enough* to manage school by myself, and my parents may not be there for me anymore, in the future. The thought that I would be left all alone helped me make the decision to become great, to become awesome, and to become an *achiever* who can prove that he is good enough.

On that day, my dad picked me up from school as he always does, to go home. Later at dinner, while at the dinner table, my dad suddenly stopped eating and fell, holding his hand on his chest, showing signs of serious pain, and struggling. I then stopped eating myself, and held my dad, asking him if he was alright. In the meantime, my mum was calling the ambulance. My dad looked at me with a blank stare in his eyes, without uttering a single word. Unfortunately, I was not able to save his life, and he shortly after, ended up dying. I was extremely upset. My Father was absolutely *everything* to me. He woke me up out of bed every morning, served me a wonderful breakfast, and drove me to school. After being taken to the hospital, the mortuary diagnostic results showed that he had a heart attack, as well as a stroke caused by heavily salted foods. He was supposed to be on a zero sodium/salt diet, due to hypertension and high blood pressure he was receiving treatment for.

Following this tragic loss, I realized my life had drastically changed, and I thought I would never be the same again. As time progressed, I was unable to go to school regularly, because my mother was not capable of supporting me. She was overweight, a diabetic, and suffering from arthritis and back complications. In addition, she was unable to support me financially for my studies. For these reasons, I dropped out of school, and joined my friends on the street. We would find cars out on the streets, and clean their windows, to earn money, to feed myself, my mother, and pay the bills. Imagine, a young boy of my age without any parents, support, or love! But I knew I had to prove that I am a big-time achiever. I needed to prove to myself that I was good enough and reinforce that I am willing do anything to survive, and make sure, that my sick mother was taken care of.

By the time I was sixteen years old, my mother's health worsened. She was admitted to the hospital, under intensive care, due to her severe medical conditions. I thought about raising some money, to assist my mother. I would walk all over the City, knocking doors in the neighborhood while holding close, a picture of my mother in her hospital bed. Soon after weeks of treatment, and my mother still lying in a hospital bed.

I remember, one Saturday morning while making breakfast for my mother, my phone rang. I looked at the caller I.D., and saw it was the on-call doctor. I frantically answered the phone and heard a very sorrowful voice...Yet another terrifying moment in my life, being in such suspense of what the doctor had called me for. The awfully dreaded time had arrived. The doctor informed me my mother had died. It was a very dark time, indeed. I became very miserable, and it so emphatically affected my life, to an extent that I had become addicted to cigarettes and alcohol. I had no control over myself, and I started eating any food that was presented to me for a form of self-medication and comfort. It did not matter whether it was junk food, fast food, or old food... I ate everything! After developing horribly bad eating habits, my health had been seriously compromised to go along. I was very overweight with a big, fat belly. I constantly suffered from body pains and muscle aches. I was sad, I was depressed, and I was at a complete loss.

In an even worse turn of events, at four o'clock in the morning one gloomy afternoon, I was found with my body lying down on the street, staring up into my friend's eyes, gasping for my air, with what felt like my soul exiting the top of my head. I had overdosed from self-medicating with cocaine, and a drinking an entire bottle of wine. As I was holding on to my precious life, the only thing on my mind was the shame of leaving this planet in this condition. The shame I was feeling in that exact moment, made me think of how my parents would have reacted, and responded to me, if they were still alive to be there for me.

In an amazing turn of events, the very next morning, I was miraculously revived. And one would think this incident would be enough to stop me from using drugs and alcohol, right? I did stop using drugs, but I continued to drink alcohol. I knew that detoxing myself was the answer, as drugs and alcohol had not solved any of my problems. The lifestyle I lived changed my vision and my goals. I would have preferred to invest my efforts into career development, rather than wasting the little income I earned, into drugs and alcohol. But, at last, I finally got the monkey off my back.

At the age of forty, I was diagnosed with type-2 Diabetes, and a few years later, became obese with high levels of cholesterol, and persistent, and unstable blood pressure. I was personally issued permanent treatment for the rest of my life as prescribed by medical doctors and specialists. I had to take Metformin twice a day, to control my blood sugar levels. Forty mg of Atorvastatin per day, to lower my cholesterol levels. I also took other medications for my elevated blood pressure, and constant back pains. Just imagine how difficult it was for me to cope with all the side effects, which never allowed me a normal life. I had no social life and suffered a total loss of confidence in myself. People insulted me, called me names like "Fat man", "Big daddy", "Shrek", and so on...Until a Nutritional specialist from a diabetic clinic advised me to go on diet, in order to start losing some weight. I was encouraged to do more physical activities, to prevent further risk of heart disease. I tried *many* diets and weight loss programs, but none of them seemed to help.

One day, I stood in front of a big mirror, and could not believe my eyes. Seeing a middle age young man, dying inside, with a big, balloon-shaped, fat belly. I was living with multiple pains throughout my body, I could not fit in nice clothes, I wore the buggy big, which is extremely difficult to find in your everyday stores. As I thought of the similarity of my parent's deaths, I looked at myself, and I realized that I absolutely had to do something to change these horrible things about myself. So, I decided to find better solutions, and make highly-positive changes to the life I had been living. It took me about five years, solely focusing on losing weight. I thought I would discover something new. I started intensively researching more weight loss programs and diet plans. I watched very many motivational videos and read plenty success stories all over the internet. And While doing this, I continued to take my medication, regularly. I happened to see an advertisement on my Facebook page, which offered a twelve-week, online training course for nutrition, how to effectively manage your weight, and live a healthy lifestyle. I took immediate action to pay and register with the course. I surprisingly had learned a lot from the course, and I also discovered so much about myself as well! I realized when I put my mind to something, and have enough passion, that I can achieve absolutely anything! I think, as well as hope, that my mother would be proud very proud of me.

The online course helped me to formulate my own diet plan. And it, in fact, has completely transformed my life! The weight loss plan has worked very well for me, as I never looked at it as a diet per say, but as a healthy way of life that allows you to feel amazing.! It is unlike any other diet I have tried before. It is not a diet, but an absolute life-changer. The full description of it will be read in proceeding chapters. Should you trust my sympathy to share this weight loss and diet plan with one in need? Well, it worked for me, as I easily lost over 130 pounds in just six months! I got back into my long-lost, fit shape, and returned to a healthy social life. I am now a very happy man, as well as healthy and fit! As I continued to lose more weight, I became far more active mentally. I am ready, and willing to venture into new endeavors.

I have maintained my bodyweight, and I now focus more on helping others to do the same, while I am now able to allow myself a more relaxed diet, as opposed to a strict diet. It has done nothing but wonders for me. Positive wonders which allow me to feel good mentally and physically. I feel better as a human being, and do not feel as if I do not fit in with the rest of society. I was freed from my struggle. I was freed from my depression. I am no longer bound to myself. Above all, I am now *totally* free from all medications. I am free from pain, Diabetes, cholesterol problems, and my once, high blood pressure is now back to normal levels. The way of life you will be taught from this book, will do the same thing for you, as it did for me...miracles. Simply put...miracles.

M ost, if not all, individuals desire to lose weight at one point or another in their lives. For many, it is done in a haphazard sort of way without much thought, planning, or time to expend. However, losing weight involves much more than determination or desire. It is necessary to implement an effective weight loss plan. Just as you would make a list for any typical household project, a structured list, in the form of a good weight loss plan is imperative, as well. There are several, key factors to formulating an effective weight loss plan. Of course, common sense would dictate that the first key factor, is to set goals. Establishing a goal is not as simple as picking a number. Setting a goal entails realistic goals, of which will not leave you feeling as though you have failed in the end. For the most part, you can plan according to your healthy weight goal that you intend to set.

A healthy weight loss goal is a starting point. It is a place where you will feel a little bit better about yourself, overall, you will be much healthier, and breathe a little bit easier. You can always continue to keep up with your weight loss goals. Setting smaller goals initially, is better than setting your sights too high, only for them to come crashing down even harder. Before anything, you must educate yourself in the field of <u>nutrition and physical activities</u>. To start your weight loss journey, think of your diet plan, identify your weight-loss goals, find your troubled areas, and personalize a weight loss plan that is suitable to you, and only you.

So, today is the day you start losing weight. I did my research and figured out how to lose weight <u>naturally</u>. I was really motivated to start putting what I learned into practice. Everything was lined up and ready. All I had to do was just to pull the trigger and get busy. It isn't going to be easy, and it isn't going to happen overnight, but, just like anything else worth having, it can be quite the journey, which rewards you with a wonderful prize, when all is said and done!

The prize, you ask. <u>A brand new</u>, fit, and trim you. Just imagine all the new clothes you will be able to buy, and how amazing you will look to others, and most importantly, yourself! You will probably kick yourself in the butt, thinking you probably should have started this process a long time ago!

When I learned how to lose weight naturally, the first thought in my head was that I was going to need to make some drastic lifestyle changes. No more pop, or overly processed foods. I was going to have to learn how to cook for myself, with all-natural ingredients, and drink a very healthy amount of water each day. Learn which foods are the most effective for weight loss, and what fluids are best to consume.

Do you happen to have a healthy cookbook? You should have one on hand, as a healthy cookbook will give you great ideas, just in case you get bored with what you are eating anytime along the way. Just remember, cookbooks are mainly suggestions, and if the recipes call for ingredients that are not a part of your overall diet plan, then simply just omit them, or substitute them for something else that your diet allows. For instance, instead of real eggs, use egg whites. Instead of sugar, use artificial sweetener.

You may have already learned to track everything you consume (food, drinks, and their calories), and to record everything in a journal. This is the easiest way to see what you are doing, keep yourself disciplined, and identify any areas you may be having difficulties keeping up with. You need to create a <u>calorie deficit</u> throughout the week, to lose the weight, you want to lose.

You need to consume less calories, or burn off 3500 calories per week, to burn more fat. Record all your activity as well, to see your improvements in lengthening the time of your daily, physical activities. Every four weeks or so, you should restructure your plan, to eliminate boredom.

If your daily meals and exercise are getting boring, you have more than likely hit a plateau (a peak, or dead end, if you will). One small change will get you back on track with your progress. So, just keep plugging away, keep losing weight naturally, and soon you will be exactly where you want to be.

I n this chapter, I am going to tell you exactly what I did in my journey, and how I did it, you will learn a step-by-step process to my weight loss journey, of which I share with you, and recommend you to follow along. It is not medically, or scientific-ally approved, but it 100% worked for me. It will work for you, as well! I will explain every single action I took all along the way. In the first week, start by deciding, as to where you must eliminate and cut off certain types of foods and beverages from your daily intake, as explained below.

Cut off _all_ sugar from your diet.

High-sugar diets contribute to prolonged elevated blood sugar, insulin resistance, and leptin resistance. All of which are linked to weight gain, and excess body fat. Although this may not be the answer you are looking for, it is true that you will lose a drastic amount of weight, simply by cutting out the sugar in your diet. On the other hand, if you continue to eat sugar, your chances of gaining weight increase drastically. The sugar in your diet, affects the amount of sugar in your bloodstream.

Studies suggest that high blood sugar levels, set up a molecular, domino-effect called _glycation_. A diet predominantly consisting of unhealthy treats can also lead to reduced skin elasticity, and premature wrinkles. Research makes it clear that excess sugar consumption and weight gain, go together. The Centers for Dis-ease Control and Prevention recommends that no more than 10 percent of your daily calorie intake should be calories from sugar. In addition to the health risks associated with eating sugar, we now know that eating more sugar inevitably means gaining more weight. If you really want to make a healthy change this year, cut-ting back on sugar is the place to start.

Research shows these types of foods are usually higher in fat, calories, cholesterol, and sodium in comparison to homemade meals. Eating too much fast food can increase risk for health problems, such as: high blood pressure, heart disease, and obesity. More specifically... The term "fast food", generally refers to food that people intend to consume quickly, either on, or off-site. There is plenty of well-researched evidence, demonstrating the various negative health effects of eating, and overeating fast food, in both the short, and long-term.

Because fast food is typically high in sugar content, salt, and saturated/trans fats, looking at the short-term effects of these nutrients can help determine what happens in the short-term, when one consumes fast food. Absolutely avoid all fried foods when you are attempting to lose weight fast. Fried foods are high in bad, saturated fats and empty calories.

Stop Eating White Bread

White bread is highly refined, and often contains a lot of added sugar. It is high on the glycemic index and can spike your blood sugar levels. It is linked to a **40% greater risk** of weight gain, and obesity. When people maintained a diet full of ultra-processed foods, they consumed more empty calories, and gained more weight. As opposed to when they maintained a diet with minimally processed foods. The results suggest the importance of identifying and eating healthy foods. Processed foods have far more bad calories, and ultimately lead to rapid fat storage in the body, and rapid weight gain. Use whole wheat bread, in place of white bread.

Diet off all fizzy drinks

Fizzy drinks can have extremely harmful effects on the body. Fizzy drinks are full of empty calories! You should absolutely avoid drinking the majority of the calories you consume. High-calorie, high-sugar soft drinks and fruit juices will destroy your fat-loss plan. They contain large amounts of sugar calories, and are easily consumed, because they are in liquid form.

Eliminate Alcohol Intake

I am not demanding that everyone stop their consumption of alcohol, but I highly advise to do so, as it did wonders for me. Alcohol consumption can often lower testosterone levels and production in men. Testosterone is a very important hormone for losing weight and gaining lean muscle. Not only does alcohol lower your inhibitions about the food choices you make, but it can also whet your appetite.

I personally stopped smoking, completely. If you stop smoking cigarettes and consuming alcohol, while making sure to exercise three times per week, you can expect to lose two to five pounds each week. Great sources of exercise include walking, cycling, swimming, and using a Treadmill (if you have one,) for 30 to 45 minutes a day.

Lower Your Sodium Consumption

Consuming too much sodium/salt can cause your body to retain more water, which will show up on the scale as extra pounds. But I am not just referring to water weight. High sodium diets appear to be linked to higher production of body fat. In particular, the kind of fat that accumulates around your midsection. Better to remove the common table salt and replace it with sea salt. Be sure to also eliminate whole milk, Cow's milk, and non-fermented dairy. Instead, a glass of skim milk is advisable once, every other day. Otherwise, you should choose non-dairy milk alternatives.

I mmediately after cutting all unnecessary foods and beverages from my diet, I started my *planned diet program.* This diet program is divided into four parts. The first part is the detox stage and during this stage you will eat mainly *fruit and vegetables* for fourteen days. It is recommended to drink at least 2.5L of water every day, to keep hydrated. Keeping hydrated will naturally suppress your appetite, and it also helps **accelerate the body's metabolism**, thus burning fat at a rapid rate. There are hundreds, maybe even thousands of recipes available for detoxing your body, but I found my own, very effective method:

Fruits and vegetables twice a day. In the morning, and before bed. A smoothie, or a mixture of green apples, cucumbers, lemon juice, and ginger with a teaspoon of honey. Blend with slightly warm water, until you have a thick, and liquid texture. When making this beverage, make enough to store throughout the week, in your refrigerator. Simply warm it up when you are ready for another!

Other Detoxing Methods:

Take a warm glass of water, and fresh Lemon. First thing in the morning, on an ***empty stomach*** to prime your pancreas, and kickstart your digestive system/metabolism. Start with one, small squeeze of lemon and gradually increase to a large squeeze to taste. The second stage of the program is where I started eating normal but selected only healthy foods. During this phase it is recommended that you eat little and eat often. This means every portion, or the quantity of food I regularly ate was, and ***must be cut in half***, to reduce the number of calories consumed. Eating this way will help to effectively boost your metabolism, which will enable you to lose weight, at a much faster rate. I added additional healthy meals which were low in fat and carbs, and high in protein.

I aimed for 600 to 700 calories per meal, along with at least 55g of carbs. Avoid white potatoes, and white pasta. Above all, I favored green vegetables, lean meats, boiled eggs, and salmon fishes. My top choices for beverages are **water and green tea**. You must include a lean protein source with every meal. Some great protein sources are lean meats, fish, eggs, low- fat cottage cheese, beans, raw nuts, raw seeds, and protein supplements. Be sure to eat protein at each meal. Snack only to take advantage of its muscle building effects.

For the first two weeks, after making all necessary changes in my diet, there was a tremendous difference I felt health-wise. I suffered from no serious side effects. I occasionally felt little headaches, nausea, and constipation. These symptoms were only a matter of my body adjusting to something new and went away quicker than I could imagine.

To curb your calorie intake, use smaller plates when eating your meals. Instead of grabbing a large dinner plate, use a smaller salad plate for each meal. It will help you control portion sizes and trick your mind into thinking you are eating much more than you are!

To enhance weight loss, chew your food carefully and thoroughly. Doing so, helps the digestion process, and allows more time for the "full" feeling to kick in. Mindful eating gives more satisfaction with less food and helps eliminate eating out of boredom.

A single bite of "forbidden" food does not have many calories, so if you can truly enjoy that one bite without needing to eat the whole thing, you will not feel so deprived. You will also be able to utilize more self-control.

In this chapter, I am going to illustrate some of my regular meals and food preparation. I would recommend you sustain a healthy diet, and lifestyle to follow, and maintain your weight.

There are many ways to prepare food, which are much healthier and leaner. Some examples of good cooking alternatives are roasting, steaming, boiling, baking, and grilling your meals. After trying some of these methods, you will not even want to eat fried food anymore.

A diet, rich in fresh fruits and vegetables, whole grains, and lean meats or other pure protein sources will help you feel satiated, while losing weight. By avoiding "fad" diets or costly, special diet foods, you can change your eating habits, become generally healthier, save money, reach your target weight goal, and maintain it easily.

If you are having trouble making your diet healthier, start by eating any food that you tend to eat at a slower pace. There are a lot of people out there who are fast eaters, so they shove down plate after plate of fatty foods, tending to overeat, before they even realize they are full. This habit leads to more calorie consumption, which is a major cause of weight gain.

Effective Meal Plans

This is my 7-day low calorie, and healthy meal preparation, which I took on the road, to lose more weight. ***Do not skip meals***, try to eat regularly to fire up your metabolism and increase more chance of losing weight.

1. Day One

Breakfast: Eat 1 bowl of Porridge

You need 75g (3 oz) of rolled oats and make according to packet instructions. Top it up with a large handful of blueberries, strawberries, or sliced peaches instead of sugar. Add up a cup of unsweetened green tea and a pot of low-fat fruit yogurt (150 ml).

Lunch: A grilled, chicken breast sandwich

You need 150 g (5 oz) of chicken breast served on barley, granary or soya bread, topped with sliced tomato and little mustard. Add up a large salad of celery, cucumber, and grated carrot. 1 banana and 10 brasil nut for snack.

Dinner: A grilled tuna steak

150 g (5 oz) of tuna topped with one serving of tomato and pepper salsa served with 100 g of new potatoes and 75g of snow pea.

2. Day Two

Breakfast: A cup of unsweetened, green tea and two slices of toast

Choose granary, barley or soya bread and spread with 2 teaspoons of ricotta cheese and 2 spoons of all fruit conserve such as blackberry. Add a pot of low-fat fruit yogurt for snack 150 g (5 oz).

Lunch: Eat a small tub of low-fat hummus

About 125 g (4 oz), served with 3 rye crispbreads and crudities of carrot, cucumber, celery, and cherry tomatoes. Add a handful of white grapes for snack 50 g (2 oz).

Dinner: Spaghetti Bolognese

Made using 75 g (3 oz) turkey or chicken mince per person, mixed with 400 g jar of ready-made, fresh tomato pasta sauce. Serve with 75 g, dry weight, of spaghetti.

3. Day Three

Breakfast: Muesli

50 g (2 oz) of any unsweetened muesli, topped with 150 ml (1/2 pint) of skimmed or soya milk. 1 apple and low frat cottage cheese for snack.

Lunch: Open tuna sandwich

Soya bread, topped with 75 g of canned tuna in brine mixed with little lemon juice and 1 teaspoon of low-fat mayonnaise, one sliced tomato and a handful of alfalfa sprouts. Add a can or carton of lentil soup 400 g. 10 almonds and 2 satsumas or kiwi fruit for snack.

Dinner: Grilled chicken breast

150 g served with 50 g of couscous (dry weight, cooked according to packed instructions) and 175 g of grilled vegetables - try a mix of auberges, red pepper, courgetti and onion.

4. Day Four

Breakfast: A bowl of noodle-shaped, bran cereal

50g, topped with 150 ml of skimmed or soya milk and 1 sliced banana. A cup of green tea with 125 g of small tub of tzatziki, served with 4 celery sticks.

Lunch: Quick Lentil salad

Mix 200 g rinsed and drained canned lentils with 75 g of lean ham, 3 chopped spring onions, 1 tablespoon of chopped parsley, a squeeze of lemon juice and season to taste. add 100 mg of blueberry smoothie mixed with 150 ml of soya milk and 150 g of soya yogurt for snack.

Dinner: Prawns with pasta

Use 150 g of prawns cooked in lemon juice and garlic.

5. Day Five

Breakfast: Omelets

Made from 1 whole egg and 3 egg whites. Fill with 50 g of grated low-fat Cheddar cheese. Serve with 1 grilled tomato. Take a glass of un-sweeter fruit juice 150 ml. Add 1 pear or apple with 25 g pumpkin seeds for snack.

Lunch: Open sandwich

made from 1 slice of granary, barley or soya bread spread with a little mustard and topped with 50 g of ham, and 50 g of cooked sliced chicken or turkey. Add sliced tomatoes, cucumber and lettuce or alfalfa sprouts.

Dinner: Steak or sole

150 g of sirloin steak or sole fillet, grilled and served with 75 g of roasted, mashed or chipped sweet potatoes and 75 g of peas.

6. Day Six

Breakfast: 1 boiled egg with 2 rye crispbreads topped with yeast extract

Serve with half a grapefruit and a smoothie made with 150 ml of skimmed milk and 4 handfuls of blueberries, strawberries, or raspberries. Add 1 slice of toast barley or soya bread and top with 1 tablespoon of peanut butter.

Lunch: Bean Salad, topped with 100 g canned tuna in spring water, 8 baby carrots and 5 cherry tomatoes. Add 1 apple or orange for snack.

Recipe: 10 minutes preparation time and 3 minutes cooking time.

75 g sliced green beans, 50 g canned red kidney beans, rinsed and drained, 25 g canned chickpeas, rinsed and drained, 1/4 onion, finely chopped 1 teaspoon of olive oil, 1 teaspoon of chopped coriander, salt, and pepper. First, cook the green beans in lightly salted boiling water for 3 minutes, then drain and refresh under cold running water. Then mix all the ingredients in a bowl and serve.

Dinner: Steak or sole

150 g of sirloin steak or sole fillet, grilled and served with 75 g of roasted, mashed, or chipped sweet potatoes and 75 g of peas.

7. Day Seven

Breakfast: Cooked breakfast

2 rashers of back bacon trimmed of all fat, grilled mushroom, grilled tomatoes, 100 g of canned baked beans and 1 slice of barley or granary toast. With a glass of skimmed milk or soya milk and 1 orange.

Lunch: Roast lunch

150 g of roast chicken, beef, or pork (no skin, crackling or other fat). Serve with 2 roast sweet potatoes, unlimited carrots, green beans, and Brussels sprouts, and 1 tablespoon of gravy. Add 2 digestive spread with a little fruit conserve.

Dinner: Grilled salmon steak

use 150 g of salmon, served with 50 g of dry egg noodles, cooked according to packed instructions, unlimited bock choy, and 1 teaspoon of sweet chili sauce. Otherwise follow recipe for preparation of salmon on noodles as below:

Preparation time is 10 minutes, plus marinating and cooked for 12 minutes.

2 skinless salmon, about 125 g each, 2table spoons of soy sauce, 1 tablespoon of dry sherry, 1 teaspoon grated fresh root ginger, 2 garlic cloves crushed, 1 tablespoon sesame oil, 2 tablespoons of water, 2 spring onions chopped, 3 tablespoons of chopped coriander leaves and 250g of dried rice noodles cooked according to packet instructions. Place the salmon on a foil-lined grill pan. Mix with two soy sauce, sherry, garlic, ginger, half of the marinade over the salmon and set aside for 10 minutes. Cook the salmon under a preheated hot grill for 5 - 6 minutes, turning it halfway through the cooking time and brushing with a little more of the marinade. heat the remaining oil in a saucepan, add the sesame seeds and spring onions and fry for 1 minute. Add the noodles and any remaining marinade to the saucepan and heat through. Serve the salmon on bed of noodles.

In addition to the above, salmon, is an excellent source of vitamin E, A and essential fatty acids that we need for healthy body. Tinned salmon also provides calcium for you, which is stored in its bones. This diet plan has been done accordingly, due to my research, after reading several books and nutritional videos. I followed it, and it worked for me, and it will work for you as well!

<u>I keep repeating the same process every week</u>. however, you may not like certain foods, but you can manage to adapt it to something else that is compatible and healthy, provided that you read ingredients and control the amount of your daily intake calories.

This diet also suggests a number of different physical activities that you could do to get the required exercise such as moving around the house doing house works, climbing or going up and down the stairs, walking for half an hour a day, cycling, swimming, playing tennis or doing some workouts. If you follow the diet but don't include exercise, then you won't see as good results as you would if you do include exercise.

This diet program is quite the effective diet program for losing weight, if you stick to it, and follow it through, including the exercises. If you are looking for a good diet program to help you lose weight, then this one may be the answer. We all know that shredding pounds of fat and losing weight in a natural way is not easy as it sounds if _you are not mentally prepared_.

It is not because of time restrictions alone, but it is also due to a fact, which people are not aware of: **"How can an individual manage losing weight naturally, by utilizing a proper diet?"** If you have time for your body, then you can easily go for a daily, small walk in the morning. You can also take a walk in the evening, which will help you to keep fit, and stress-free.

Y ou have built up the courage to start finding ways to lose weight rapidly. It is now time to act, and finally become the person you have always dreamed of being! There is absolutely no room for, or reason to hesitate from becoming a better person. You have the guide to rapidly burning body fat, right at your fingertips! Simply follow this guide, be patient, and watch the results unfold as you have always wanted them to.

www.ingramcontent.com/pod-product-compliance
Lightning Source LLC
Chambersburg PA
CBHW051145250726
48655CB00007B/3253